# A Newbies Guide to Travel Nursing

By

## Kay (Epstein LaRue) Slane, RN, CGM
(Certificate of Grad-level Management)

A Newbies Guide to Travel Nursing

© Kay Slane, RN, CGM
aka… Epstein LaRue

Edited by Caroline Heywood
Interior Design by: Kay Slane
Cover Design by Kay Slane

Published in April 2018
Printed in the United States of America

A Highway Hypodermics, LLC Book
http://highwayhypodermics.com/

Idaho, U.S.A.

*Dedicated to:*

*All the travel nurses that belong to my Facebook Group:*
*Travel Nursing Newbies*

# INTERIOR CONTENTS:

# FOREWORD

# The Travel Healthcare Lifestyle

Travel nursing can be a very lucrative career both financially and personally. This is not just a job, but a way of life. When I first began to think about travel nursing, there were a few websites that gave me some tips on how to get started, but for the most part, I was at the mercy of the travel companies to provide me with the information. I didn't have anyone to tell me NOT to give my phone number out to 20 travel companies, because my phone wouldn't stop ringing. 12 years later, there are a plethora of publications, websites, and social media communications to keep you updated.

This little guide brings to the new travel nurse what he or she needs to know - to get them started - in a small compact package. It will guide you through the necessary steps to arm yourself with the tools that will not only let you be a travel nurse but which will also allow you to excel as a travel nurse. It is a summary of the main ideas that you should consider.

When you are ready to delve deeper into travel nursing and the finer aspects, I encourage you to purchase Highway Hypodermics: Travel Nursing 2017 by Epstein Larue, Joseph C. Smith, and Aaron Highfill.

# CHAPTER ONE

## *WHEN CAN I GO INTO TRAVEL NURSING?*

One of the most common questions that I see on social media is, "When can I go into travel nursing?"

Graduating nursing school is a life event that will always stay with you. All the years of hard work and sacrifice are finally over, and you are ready to make a difference in people's lives by providing excellent nursing care. However, as many a seasoned nurse can testify, you will realize that things are different in the real world compared to the relative comfort experienced in nursing school. In school, you worked closely with qualified staff and instructors. Now, that support network has changed, leaving you with the task of developing your advanced skills more autonomously.

If you have an excellent preceptor who will help you develop those skills, you will be well on your way to achieving what it takes to be a successful travel nurse.

During nursing school, you learned the basics of nursing, including how to complete a head-to-toe assessment, taking a set of vitals, putting in a Foley catheter, drawing blood, the correct way to give medications, and how to start IVs. During your first year as a qualified nurse, depending on the unit on which you are working, you will have opportunities for advanced nursing skills including starting difficult IVs, accessing port-a-caths, maintaining arterial lines, and perhaps even management of a ventilator.

During this first year, you will also work on caring for many patients with minimal supervision. You will develop your critical thinking skills along with making crucial judgments that can affect patients' lives. These abilities are not handed to you during your first year. The knowledge is obtained through on-the-job training and personal development - every day you should be learning something new.

One potential obstacle in personal development is the tendency for newly qualified nurses to feel that their superiors are out to catch them. It couldn't be further from the truth. During your first years out of school, you are building on those valuable and essential experiences and the senior, more experienced staff want to help you become as confident as they appear to be. The reality is that everyone is learning all the time – it never stops. So they are not out to 'eat the young' but, instead, are there to support you in that transition period.

For those nurses who want to be a traveling nurse in their first year, this type of frustration can increase because your future employer hopes that you will have that confidence to perform those skills that you have been taught. If you find yourself in a challenging situation, it is important to remember that your employer's duty is, first of all, to the safety of the patients. If you think that you will require the cushioning protection for a while longer after completion of nursing school, it would be wise to reconsider travel nursing as a prospect until you have some experience in a stable job. On the other hand, you may be lucky to find an employer who is more sympathetic to the needs of a 'newbie', and the advantage of global communication via the Internet is that this type of information can be discovered much more easily these days.

A new graduate who has already gained experience as a Licensed Practical Nurse (LPN), has some of this necessary 'know-how'. So while he or she may be a newly graduated RN, that previous experience will have provided the person with enough time to accommodate him or herself to the experience of working with less direct supervision. Still, I might advise an RN with previous LPN experience to wait six months – this should, of course, be a personal decision based on the individual. Situations can still arise where, out of the blue, you are in a position of having to defend your actions, and it may seem that nobody is there to back you up. The state board, like the employer, puts patient safety first.

For practical reasons, there are a few travel nursing companies who do hire newly qualified graduate nurses. So, do your homework and if you think that you have what it takes – go for it!

For any brand-new graduate going from nursing school into travel nursing, I would think about it. I would not want a mistake to happen, and soon you find yourself in front of the state nursing board related to the fact that you thought you knew exactly what you were doing. And, I can guarantee you that the Travel Company, recruiter, and hospital nursing manager will not be standing there with you. You've been in school for years, please don't give up that license in your first year. We firmly suggest that you have at least two years of experience/

For helpful insights on what to expect during your first year as a new graduate, I would also highly recommend, "The Everything New Nurse Book" by Kathy Quan, RN. As she states, "Nursing is one of the most challenging professions, both emotionally and physically, but it is also one of the most rewarding." This book is designed to help you understand your role as a new nurse and how to take care of yourself so you can enjoy a long and exciting career taking care of patients.

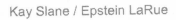

# CHAPTER TWO

## *What Travel Agencies Want In a Travel Nurse*

As an author and travel nurse, I have spent the last 15 years making every attempt to bridge the gap between travel nursing agencies and nurses.

In those 11 years, I have come to know quite a few experienced recruiters. I recently reached out to some of the most experienced nurses, and one 'newbie,' to see what they looked for in a new traveling nurse.

The first criterion I found is determining what type of hospital the nurse is at and what kind of qualifications they have according to their specialty. Lauren from Cirrus Medical Staffing states, "Having certifications such as BLS, ACLS, TNCC, CEN, CCRN, and AWHONN is very important to a hospital along with where the nurse's experience is from. Were they at a teaching hospital? What was trauma level the hospital? New nurses who only have a short time of hospital or critical access experience are harder to place to meet the requirements of the employing hospital".

The second is that nurses need to know what hospitals are usually looking for. I encourage nurses to start researching graduation and start connecting with other travel nurses to gain as much knowledge as possible. As a result of that research, they will probably discover that "most hospitals require nurses to have 1 to 2 years of experience so that they can hit the ground running", states Nathan from TotalMed Staffing.

The third criterion is that any new nurse needs to be open to hearing information. Crystal from Expedient Medstaff states, "The first time traveler needs to develop an idea of what Travel Nursing is by doing a lot of research. They need to have an idea of the bill rate and how that 'pie' is distributed to the travel nurse and the travel company. Candidates need to listen to experienced travelers to get an idea of the reality of Travel Nursing. It is not always fun; there are plenty of rough times!"

The fourth criterion is that travelers should try to know what they want to do with their nursing career. Richard, from 24/7 MedStaff, explains, "New traveling nurses need to know and understand: what they are going to specialize in, their shift preferences, what compliance documents will be required and how to submit them promptly, what free days they require, and finally, their budgetary needs. Concerning qualities, a good travel nurse needs to be flexible, have great communication skills, be honest, and be able to commit to the duration of an assignment."

The fifth criterion is that you need to do an honest assessment of your skills and choose a reliable recruiter who will review your skills checklist and give you a candid assessment. "If a nurse is not honest with me then we are just wasting our time. The market has changed significantly, and it changes pretty swiftly. If the nurse is willing to go to a less sought after location, a year of experience in that field is usually acceptable. They also need to be aware that if they are looking to go into a highly competitive market where there are nurses with 5+ years' of experience, there is no guarantee they will get a position," states Vinny of Core Medical Group.

Lastly, it is essential to find a great recruiter who will help you along the way. "Some companies will throw you into any job without caring about whether or not it is a good fit for your skill set because it is all about them making money. It's like randomly testing your macaroni to see if it's done by throwing it against the cabinet to see if it sticks. There are so many different variables to consider if travel nursing could be right for you. Do your research online, and ask lots of questions," states Holly with Fusion Medical Staffing.

So to review, the top six things that agencies look for in a new traveling nurse include:

The nurse needs to determine what specialty she wants to invest in according to the hospital that she has come from and what certifications she has.

The nurse needs to know what hospitals are usually looking for.

The nurse needs to be open to hearing information and do a lot of research.

The nurse needs to know what they want to do with their nursing career.

The nurse needs to do an honest assessment of their skills and choose a recruiter who will review the skills checklist and give you a candid assessment.

The nurse needs to find a great recruiter who will help you along the way.

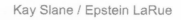

# CHAPTER THREE

## *The Physical Aspects of Travel Nursing*

The biggest question I want you to ask yourself is, "Why do I want to travel?"

If you are traveling for the money, then you are going to find that travel nursing can be very lucrative, but none of us are making a million dollars a year doing this. You'd like to travel to see the United States. Perhaps you're ready for a new home base. Or you think that you'd like to live in Colorado.

The adventure of travel nursing is gratifying, but it isn't always roses; there can be some huge thorns out there too. If not taken very seriously, and if you're not honest with an assessment of your skills, then you can find yourself in front of a board of nursing trying to explain why a patient died as a result of improper nursing care. If that happens, I can guarantee you that the director of nursing, the charge nurse, your recruiter, your staffing company, and other nurses are NOT going to be standing by you while you defend yourself. I cannot stress enough how important it is for you to be physically and mentally ready for travel nursing!

How do you know if you are physically ready to go? First, we will look at your nursing skills, and make an honest assessment of your readiness for work and your commitment.

As a travel nurse, you will be required to fill out a skills checklist before your first assignment when you change companies and on an annual basis. This is a list of nursing skills that you may be required to perform while on assignment. This includes your assessments skills and intervention skills. Can you correctly insert a Foley catheter or an IV? How often do you perform that skill: weekly, monthly, or less often? There are usually 3 to 4 pages listing these skills on which you will rate yourself concerning how frequently you perform these skills, and how proficient you are. Have you ever performed the skills? Are you moderately experienced and may still require a resource person? Are you proficient and can perform them independently, or are you an expert and don't mind teaching that skill? As a traveling nurse, you need to be proficient in about 80% of what is on the skills checklist. If you checked off more than 20% of those skills which you have either never carried out or for which you still require supervision, you need to think twice about travel nursing - you MUST be able to work on your own without too much support or supervision!

How organized are you? How up-to-date is your résumé? You must have a current résumé to apply to any travel nursing company. Do you have all your immunizations and your titers ready to go? I have not been on a travel assignment yet that didn't want my Hepatitis B, MMR, and Varicella titers. Make sure that you have all your pertinent medical records ready to go. What about other certificates? Your unit specific certificates, such as BLS, ACLS, PALS, TNCC, STABLE & AWHONN all need to be up to date.

And, are you ready to commit to staying at a hospital for 13 weeks? In my 11 years, I have been lucky in only having two assignments in which I counted down the days before finishing.

The ONLY reason that a travel nurse should leave an assignment is if your license is in danger. Family members become sick and even pass away while you're on assignment. A lot of hospitals will let you have bereavement time off by taking a week off, but chances are, you will have to add a week to your contract. As the travel nurse can you handle multiple admits, discharges, and have the sickest patients on the floors? Can you handle all four of your patients being in isolation for VRE, MRSA, TB and Neutropenic Precautions?

# CHAPTER FOUR

## *The Mental Aspects Of Travel Nursing*

One of the most common questions that I see on social media is, "When can I go into travel nursing?"

One of the biggest parts of being a travel nurse is being flexible and adaptable to new situations. I have witnessed a large number of nurses asking if they can put "no floating" in their contract. Well, yes, you can put that in your contract, but I don't see many hospitals accepting that. Part of being a travel nurse is being flexible and floating to other floors on which you are competent to work. Perhaps not so fortunately for less experienced nurses, many hospitals hire ICU nurses who are personnel with more advanced skills. They are competent to work on any floor of the hospital, and so they are more employable. This does create a problem for other potential recruits because ICU nurses are used to taking care of 2 to 3 patients at a time. It is not ideal, but it does happen, and you should be flexible to work on any floor for which you are competent.

Can you "hit the floor running?" Travel nurse assignments are never alike. Sometimes you get 4 hours of orientation; at other times you will get four days of orientation. As a travel nurse you must remember that irrespective of where you are working, the basic nursing process never changes. Your job is to assess, plan, implement, and then evaluate. The one thing that does change is how you get from point A to point B. There are several ways to accomplish a task, and a useful piece of advice is, "When in Rome, do as the Romans." Yes, you have to perform tasks the way you were taught, but keep in mind that there may be several ways to get the same thing done.

Adapting to new floors is another responsibility of a traveling nurse. You must use an arsenal of strategies to be able to float from one floor to the next. Again, we go back to the basics of nursing. You need to assess, plan, implement, and then evaluate what worked and did not work for that patient. With floating, you may need to use another nurse's assessment and evaluations to implement your plan. This is called teamwork and adapting to new situations. As a traveler, your critical thinking skills must be sharp, intact, and ready to fire at any moment. You cannot sit back and see what someone else is going to do; you must step forward and become a patient advocate.

Part of the 'high' of travel nursing for a genuine travel nurse is stepping into a world of the unknown. It is exciting for us to go into a strange hospital, in a strange town and maybe even in a state to which we have never been. Some of the anxiety of going to a new assignment can be relieved by doing our research on the new assignment. That is the great thing about internet forums, chat rooms, and groups - you can network with other nurses who might have been at the same hospital or city. Research can be fun! In fact, I'm in that stage of an assignment now. I was recently submitted to a hospital in central California. My husband and I have spent HOURS on the computer looking for recreational vehicle (RV) parks and fun things to do in central California. By going to www.homefair.com, we have discovered that our next assignment is in a town with a population of 35,000, mostly a Caucasian population (70%), with an average household income of 89,000. The general public has a high school diploma, with 30% having completed college. The high temperatures range from 57 to 98 degrees with the low temperatures ranging from 73 to 36 degrees (not quite freezing!). Even more impressive is that we found that the crime rate is an '85', which is lower than the 100 marker - the average for the United States.

One of the inevitable facts of travel nursing is that we have to leave our home. Depending on current situations this can be a good or bad feature. The one great thing about travel nursing is that you can be closer to family in a time of need, but you can also be farther. In 2004, I was lucky to be a travel nurse when my father was diagnosed with Guillain Barre Syndrome. I could find an assignment close to my parent's house in Oklahoma, while my house was in Idaho. On the other hand, another traveler friend of mine had to travel 2000 miles back home to bury his father.

The last variable that you need to evaluate before embarking on a travel nursing career is taking a long look at how much stability you require. Can you tolerate moving around every three months?  Do you get bored and would like to move around more often?  Or perhaps you prefer some stability and would, ideally, renew your assignments?  I belong to the latter category, and so I love to renew contracts. In fact, at my last hospital, I renewed three times for a total of 51 weeks. The magical thing about travel nursing is that you don't have to do that; you can go to a different place every three months!

One less attractive feature of this method of job-seeking is that recruiters come and go.  Ask any travel nurse, and they will tell you that your recruiter can make or break any assignment.  As a traveling nurse, can you tolerate the possibility of your recruiter leaving in the middle of an assignment?  You would in that situation be given the task of trusting someone new with some of your career decisions.

Travel nursing can be a fun and exciting career, but it also can be your downfall.  Through this series of articles, I truly hope that I have stimulated some brain cells, allowing you to make a competent decision on whether travel nursing is the perfect choice for you!

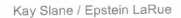

# CHAPTER FIVE
## *Doing Your Research*

Now that you have your list of benefit requirements use the up-to-date graph, "The Ultimate List of Travel Companies," on the website www.highwayhypodermics.com to get an idea of which companies offer the benefits that are most important to you.

By looking at 'Travel Company Information', you will find the benefits list, plus a lot more information on companies including evaluations, company profiles, and recruiter profiles.

Do more research on the Internet by visiting discussion boards and travel nursing forums, and ask other nurses what they think of those travel companies. This is where you will discover the inside information on these companies. However, be aware that travel companies may well have their representatives contributing to these forums – use pertinent questions to make sure you're getting an unbiased opinion.

After narrowing your decision down to about five different companies that you would like to work for, submit a complete application for employment to these five companies.

Upon receiving your application, a recruiter will promptly contact you. Talk to the recruiter and find out what hospitals they have that you are interested in. Find out how many jobs they have available for your specialty. This is especially important if you have a specialty that is on the 'hard to find' list, such as psychiatric, rehabilitation, or pediatric emergency care nursing.

Not only should the recruiter interview you, but you should also interview the recruiter! This is done most easily if you get out a notebook to keep track of the questions that you have asked.

Each entry should list the company's name, address, phone number, and the person you talked to.

The next entry should be the size of the company. While smaller companies may not provide a large selection of places to travel to, the customer service is usually impeccable.

Next, you might want to know what kind of structure their recruiters work with. If the recruiters work on a commission basis, there is a greater chance of a recruiter wanting to sign you up for personal financial gain. If a company recruits by a shared commission, you are more likely to find a company for whom teamwork is foremost - to the advantage of the travel nurse. In summary, some companies cater to the hospital, whereas others cater to the nurse.

You will also want to know what the process is in case you decide to change recruiters. When problems arise, you want a recruiter that you feel you can work with. If you feel like the recruiter isn't working with you, or if there are personality clashes, it is much easier to switch recruiters than to switch companies. You don't want to get attached to a company that is not going to work with you on problem-solving. Along with this, you also need to find out if there is a recruiter supervisor and who it is. Sometimes this will be the owner in a small company or a regional supervisor in a larger company.

You will want to know from the recruiter if they can place you regionally, nationally, or internationally. Some companies only cover certain regions, or they have different offices for different regions. Some companies only cover certain states, and there are some states that are only contracted with certain companies. If you are interested in traveling internationally, you will want to find a company that specializes in international travel. International travel brings into play a very different set of rules because of immunizations, passports, work visas, etc.

You will want to know how many assignments are available with the company. This is especially important if a location is your number one priority. If this requirement isn't fulfilled, then you are going to find yourself hunting for a different company for each assignment.

You will need to find out what kinds of specialties are provided for by the company. The most common specialty companies that I have found are companies who specialize only in providing hospital operating room personnel. A few companies out there specialize only in providing management personnel. If your specialty is med-surg nursing, you will have quite a few companies to choose from; but if your specialty is psychiatric or rehabilitation nursing, you might have trouble finding a company who provides those types of jobs.

I also advise that you keep a note of priority benefits. Your priority benefit list might include: the name of the insurance company and the type of insurance provided, and whether it's a PPO, HMO, or just a major medical plan. What are the deductibles and how much does the insurance cost the travel nurse? Yes, there are companies out there who provide free medical insurance for their travel nurses. This is a question that you have to ask yourself: are you willing to pay a small amount for your insurance?

You will want to know when you will be paid and how you will be paid. Most companies will send you a weekly check, but there are some out there that only pay bi-weekly or monthly. If you receive a housing stipend, find out if you will be paid the stipend on a weekly or monthly basis. Are monthly stipends paid at the first of the month or the end of the month?

You will probably want to find out if the company writes guaranteed hours into their contracts. How many hours do you want to work? Some companies will give you a guarantee of thirty-six hours, while others will guarantee you forty-eight hours. Are those hours broken into eight-hour shifts, ten-hour shifts, or twelve-hour shifts?

What length of assignment does the company offer? In a fast response situation, you might find assignments lasting only four weeks. At other places, you might find companies that offer six to nine-month contracts. For those nurses who are traveling with school-age children, maybe a nine-month contract during the school year would be preferred over a short-term contract.

If you are considering your accommodation needs, you will want to know what type of housing is available. Are there are any additional costs to the traveler? Will you have to share housing with another traveler? If you take the subsidy, you will want to know if they pay just what your expenses are, or if you get to keep any of the extra money should there be some left over after paying your expenses. The housing subsidy should be equal to the cost of renting a one-bedroom apartment.

Another thing that you might want to know in the company interview is if airfare and rental car fees are provided. This is especially true if you plan to travel somewhere outside the continental forty-eight states, such as Hawaii, Alaska, or the Virgin Islands. While airfare is needed for a trip to Hawaii, some travel nurses opt out of the rental car fees and purchase a vehicle from other travel nurses who are leaving the island.

# CHAPTER SIX

## *Finding the Right Travel Company*

There are plenty of travel companies out there. Do your shopping; do not just grab the first one that makes you an offer.

Plan to start looking for a company about a month before starting work if at all possible. This process will include finding out more about benefits, locations, and general operations of the travel company.

When shopping around for a travel nursing company, be aware that some are going to want you to fill out their application and send all of your records and qualifications before they will submit you to a hospital. At this point, be careful to give them just your basic information and let them know that you are just shopping for a travel company. Don't make the mistake of filling out applications and checklists for fifty different companies just to interview them.

Also, be careful about who you give your phone number to until you have done your homework. Once you give the travel company your phone number, you will receive phone calls every thirteen weeks, asking you about assignments. It won't be long before those minutes on your cell phone have been used up.

After reading this, you will be able to find the one company that is going to make you happy in the long run and which goes where you want to go. But first, we need to begin the process of narrowing down your choices.

One thing that should be on that list is your wage requirements. Do you have to have over $30-35 or can you survive on $25 per hour? Know exactly what you need—and not necessarily what you want—to live your new lifestyle.

What kind of housing do you require? Are you single and fancy-free? Is a motel or extended-stay sufficient? The positives of staying in a motel are that they usually have laundry facilities, a pool, and of course, maid service!

Most companies will provide a one-bedroom furnished apartment. You just bring clothes, linens, and personal items. Watch this option, though, because some companies will tell you that you have a 'private' bedroom when in reality you have a private bedroom with shared common areas with another traveler. This may be fine for a lonely traveler, but many of us like the privacy of our apartment. This option does not work out if you travel with your family.

Planning to take your family? Most companies will work with you on that. They will provide a two-bedroom apartment for you, although you may be expected to pay utilities or some of the rent.

Another option if you are traveling with your family is to become full-time RVers. This becomes a bit more complicated if you are a female traveler. Not that you can't do it by yourself with a trailer or a 5th wheel, but I would suggest getting a motorhome. Motorhomes are much easier to move and to park.

As a full-time traveling family, you have the option of your children changing school every three to six months, or you can travel according to the school year. Homeschooling is becoming more and more popular and worth looking into. In a later chapter, I will discuss the subject of housing and what to do before your first assignment.

What are you location requirements? Do you want to stay in your home state or the surrounding states? With the invention of compact states, you could decide just to travel in compact states. Favorite destinations seem to be Hawaii and Alaska on the west coast in the winter, or Maine in the summer and winter in Florida for the east coast. You might even choose to stay in the middle by going to North Dakota in the summer and to Texas in the winter.

Love to ski? Then go snow skiing in Colorado in the winter and the lakes of Tennessee for water skiing in the summer. The possibilities are endless.

What about other benefits, such as health insurance, 401K, continuing education requirements, longevity, and completion bonus? These things all matter in your decision!

Find the one company which has the appropriate nursing retention program. What kinds of benefits are added on, the longer that you are with them? Almost all companies have this, whether it is instead of money or fits into a reward program.

Don't settle for a company that does not provide a 401K program. Not only should they allow you to put tax-free money in, but they should also be making some kind of vested contribution.

Make sure that the company is reliable. Once you get 'out there' in the big world of travel nursing, there are going to be days where the only friend you have is your recruiter or staffing supervisor.

Keep your list handy in your planning stage. As we explore your career more as a travel nurse, you may want to add more ideas. Don't forget to add to your list the places where you would like to travel. You will need that information because not all travel companies go to all areas of the United States and beyond.

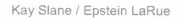

# CHAPTER SEVEN
## *Finding the Right Location*

If location is the most important thing to you, you will need to find the travel company that goes where you want to go.

For example, if you want to travel to a hospital in Arizona, you would first find companies that are approved for Arizona contracts. (There are some states and some job registries where only a select number of companies can retain those positions, such as the Arizona Hospital Association.) To find out this information, look on the Internet for the Arizona Hospital Association, go to the website and find the list of companies that provide for the staffing needs in Arizona.

The next step is investigating the hospital and community that you are looking at. Search the Internet for more information. Search area chats rooms and searches for a messaging program for people in that area. The Chamber of Commerce, City Website, and Craigslist are good places to start.

The best place I have found to gain information about a new location is at http://www.homefair.com/. It is here that you can find information on a cost-of-living comparison, city report, school reports, crime statistics, moving calculator, choosing the right school, and rental furniture. The first place that I start is with the city report. This will give you a good idea of what to expect regarding crime rate, city size, climate, age demographics, and the major employers.

Other useful information that you can find here is the average rent for an apartment and what to expect in salary from the salary calculator.

Another excellent source for information is on http://www.apartment.com/. This is especially useful if you are assisting a company in obtaining your housing. You can also compare what your company is setting you up in, compared to other housing available in that area.        You     can     also     check     out www.apartmentratings.com to see if there is anyone happy with the place.   Just remember to read the comments and don't necessarily go by the rating. Another thing to remember is that people who are upset are more likely to post a rating than a person who is happy with the place.

This brings up another critical element in choosing a travel company: look at, and ask about, the type of housing each company provides in the area that you are looking at.  A lot can be told about a company by their housing.  Are you getting a deluxe company with a deluxe apartment, or are you getting an older shack?

The companies who care about their nurses know that a nurse will only be happy if they feel comfortable and safe in their surroundings.   Get to know your surroundings online before accepting any job assignment!

Find out what amenities are available in the apartment or motel.  Do they have a pool or spa?  What about a workout or weight room?  Do they allow pets, and if so, how much does it cost for a pet deposit?

If you travel in a recreational vehicle, you want to find out if there are any RV parks close by that accept long-term visitors. I am finding out now that some of the newer parks will only accept you if your vehicle was made in the last ten years.

I work nights, and my husband is disabled; therefore, our two main priorities are a hot tub and a place that is quiet during the day.

If you have a child, you might want to find out about what schools are available or what support systems are available for home-schooled children. I also want to know where the local church is and what kind of teen program they have.

Now that we have a company and an area that we would like to go to, the next critical step is to investigate and interview the hospital.

Ask yourself, "What type of hospital am I looking for?" Do you prefer a large hospital, a teaching hospital, or a smaller community hospital? Or...does size matter?

Are you looking to go to a specific region in the country? Make a list of what you are looking for in a hospital. Even though I came from a small hospital, I enjoyed my time at the level one trauma center that I worked at in Phoenix, Arizona.

Yes, I was more stressed out, but I was treated as a name and a number. I had a large support system there, which helped out also. Most importantly, I learned that although I prefer a smaller facility, I should not be afraid of a larger facility.

Get out another piece of paper and take notes on your hospital interviews. Keep the notes of all your interviews together in a folder or on a clipboard. If a nurse manager brings up something that you hadn't thought of, add that to your list.

Always know the exact location of the hospital. Know what area of town the hospital is in. Then use that information to check out the crime rate of the hospital area.

I might consider working in a higher crime rate area, but I would not want to live there. Do you have a "high crime" plan of action? My husband would be taking me to work and picking me up. I would much prefer to work in an area of low crime, but the amenities of a bigger hospital and town might be worth the 13-week assignment.

For example, I looked at going to a suburb of Los Angeles. This was after I had spent 13 weeks in Phoenix. No, I wasn't too thrilled about staying and working in a place like that, but the amenities were the reason I would spend 13 weeks there. I would love to take my son to all the sights around Los Angeles, such as Disneyland and Universal Studios.

What system do I use? I call it my "Glendale" system! While working in Northern Phoenix, I lived in the Glendale area. This was about as much crime as I would ever want to get into. So, when I'm looking for a place to go, I always compare it to the Glendale, Arizona crime rate. Maybe you would want to use your hometown as a measure.

# Chapter Eight

# *Finding the Right Hospital & Unit*

How big is the unit will you be working on? How many nurses are on duty? What is the nurse-to-patient ratio? Depending on the number of patient and nurses, the charge nurse is also required to take patients. This affects the amount of time they are going to have to assist you if needed.

Do they have licensed vocational/practical nurses and certified nursing assistants? It makes a big difference if you are a registered nurse and not only have all of your patients to take care of but you also have to take care of all the intravenous medications of another nurse.

Think of unit specific questions also. In the intensive care unit you might want to know the average number of ventilators, how many surgical patients, how many medical patients, or how many cardiac patients are there.

As an emergency room nurse, I would want to know if nursing or respiratory therapy does the electrocardiograms. I want to know if I have an emergency room tech to assist me with dressings and splints. Am I responsible for my lab draws, or do the lab techs come to the emergency room and draw?

In this technology and information age, you might want to know what kind of charting is done. Do they chart on paper or the computer? Do they have care plan problem charting or subjective, objective, assessment, and plan charting?

What about the medical system? Do they have a computerized system like a pyxis? How do I obtain medications "after hours"? The time it takes for you to get that medication may be a little slower if you have to have the house supervisor get the medication, or if the hospital has a 24-hour pharmacist available.

How often do the nurses float and what area would you be expected to float to? Tell them up front if there are any floors that you would not be willing to work on.

Next, you will need to know about meals. This is especially true if you work nights. At the small hospitals, the night shift is usually responsible for bringing their supper, but in one place where I worked the night shift received their meals free. Plates of food were left in the refrigerator, and we just warmed them up in the microwave at break time. At the larger facility that I worked at, the cafeteria was open for an hour or two.

The next thing that I can think of to ask would be about special uniforms or the color of uniforms. I worked in one nursing home where the nursing assistants wore colors, and the medication nurses wore a different color. The charge nurses could wear colored pants, but we had to always wear white tops because the elderly associated "white" with a professional nurse.

Next, you might want to ask about the town, although you should have done some homework on the town already. What is the population? Do they have a seasonal fluctuation?  In central California, I worked in a small city in which they had a great influx during the harvest season.  During that time of the year, it was also very difficult to find a place to live.

What is the average temperature for the time that you are going to be there?  Do they have four actual temperature ranges and seasons, or just hot, hotter, hell, and whew, I can breathe again!  Is it cold, colder, polar bear, then a few months of defrost?  Personally, I'm trying to get this snowbird thing worked out... north in the summer and south in the winter!

# Chapter Nine

## *Getting Your Documents in Order*

You've talked to the hospital, and now you are ready to head off to your new destination. Our recruiter talks to the hospital and the deal is done on their end, but what about the deal on your end?

This is where things get fun. This lovely document, my friend, is called a "contract" or an "agreement." Everything is settled upon verbally; then the contract is drawn up and sent to you. Your first assignment before you get to your destination is to read the fine print of the document that will dictate what your career will be like for the next 13 weeks.

Negotiations with the recruiter can sometimes be a tedious job, but every detail must be dealt with. Your first indication might be to think, "We discussed everything, and it's in there." No! I guarantee you that the first time you do that will be the last time that you do that. I have yet to have a contract that I didn't have to add something to.

Sit down in a quiet place and read your contract, word for word and between the lines. If there is any part that you do not agree with, or have questions about, do not sign it until those questions have been answered.

If you have a vacation planned, or if you need certain days off, make sure that you get those dates in writing. It has been my experience that if it is not in writing, you may have to just live with the consequences. If it is in writing, you are guaranteed those days off.

When you open up your new-hire packet, you will find several pages of legal jargon that state that you are going to a hospital or facility to work for a certain amount of time for a certain dollar amount. It says that you are going to act like a professional and that the client-hospital and your travel company are going to treat you like a professional.

The employment relationship is the legal arrangement of the contract. As a staff nurse, you were used to being an "at-will" employee, which means that your continued employment was at the discretion of you and the hospital. As a travel nurse, you will become a "contracted employee." Yes, they can still let you go, but as a contracted employee they are obligated to compensate you for breach of contract.

Another type of relationship between nurse, hospital, and agency is called "match-hire," in which the nurse is matched to the hospital, but the nurse is paid directly by the hospital. In this situation, the agency matches you to the hospital. The hospital not only gives you a regular paycheck, but they give the agency a preset dollar amount for your services. Be careful of this situation, because benefits can be very tricky here. The agency can't give you certain benefits because you don't get a regular paycheck from them, and the hospital doesn't give you benefits because you aren't a full-time employee. This situation can cause further confusion between nurse and travel agency when it comes to longevity benefits.

We all should know our professional responsibilities, but because some nurses do not act professionally at all times, those paragraphs have to be added. This part of the contract states that if you cannot show up for your assignment, then you need to call at least two hours before your shift starts. This section also draws the lines of when you, in effect, "voluntarily quit." Although some companies allow for a "lenient" day, most of the time, if you do not show up for the first day, they consider that a voluntary quit. As a protection to the travel company, a clause is added that states that if you act carelessly, that affects patients or the client hospital, you can and will be turned into the local authorities and state nursing board.

The professional responsibility section is also where you agree to follow the standards set up by The Joint Commission. (TJC), the Occupational Health & Safety Organization (OSHA), and the Nurse Practice Act. This section also includes the fact that you must keep your credentials and licenses that are required for the assignment current. These include documentation that might be needed relating to your nursing qualifications, including ACLS, PALS, TNCC, and State Licenses.

Next, you will find your start date, the end date, the facility to which you are assigned, your shift, your on-call time, and your flexibility or floating capabilities. This section might also include whether or not you have guaranteed hours.

If you do not want to float or do not want to be put on call, then make sure that is put into writing. If you do not feel comfortable floating to a certain floor, like O.B. or O.R., then state that in your contract. When reviewing this section of your contract, you also must be mindful that part of a travel nurse's job is to be flexible. This is your contract, and you must protect yourself!

Your travel arrangements and lodging arrangements should be next. Listed here will be your permanent home address and even your temporary address. If applicable, your travel housing stipend amount should also be listed here.

When it comes to your work salary and housing, get everything in writing, and don't ever take anything for granted. If there are days off that you want to be guaranteed, ask for them in your contract. If floating is a possibility, specify the situations that you will not float; as in the fact that "I don't feel comfortable in ICU or OB," so you put in your contracts that you will not float to ICU or OB. If you want every weekend on or every weekend off or you're willing to work every other weekend, specify that in your contract if that matters to you. Put it in writing whether you wish to work overtime or not.

If there is to be any deduction in pay related to a missed shift that should also be included. If you are put on call, these deductions should not apply. Make sure that the on-call stipulations are there in the contract.

Included also might be what you are to be paid for a per diem rate. This rate is a fixed rate that is paid to you for food, parking, and other ancillary expenses that you will incur while away from your home state. As of writing this chapter, the maximum allowed by the government is no more than $30 per day. Taxes should be taken out of your hourly rate, but not out of your per diem rate. Companies most often call this a "tax-advantage" program. You will file your taxes in your home state and will get back most of the money that you paid into another state, but also expect to pay your state taxes.

It will also indicate what is included in your housing arrangements. With some companies, you will also pay for cable and local phone, but most of them will not pay for those extra utilities. But then again, everything is negotiable in this business!

You cannot get paid unless you turn in your time slips. These time slips are usually faxed to the company that you are contracted with. Some companies have you also mail the original to them, while other companies have you give a copy to the nursing manager. If a company wants certain information on this form, it is also included in this part of the contract.

The last part of the contract might include more legal jargon about benefits, injury on the job, alcohol use, illegal drug use, and the confidentiality clause. All of these important items are included in your contract to protect both you and the company.

In fact, that is the sole purpose of any contract that you have with any company: it is to protect you, the employee, and the company. In this business, verbal agreements mean nothing. Have you ever watched those court shows in the afternoon? Always, the judge wants to know if you had it in writing. If it isn't in writing, you just lost. A nice recruiter may be a pleasure to work with, but just remember that they are working for the money they get from handling your contract. Remember, they are no more than nursing salespeople.

# Chapter Ten
## *And You Are Off!*

After you have picked out the hospital and travel company, you need to prepare for the next assignment. The company will send you another employee packet with many official forms that need to be filled out: forms required by the Occupational Health and Safety Authority, the Internal Revenue Service, and other miscellaneous company forms.

You then need to make sure that your living arrangements and transportation arrangements are all squared away. The travel company usually makes flight arrangements, but you also need to arrange for your items to get there. Can you get everything in three suitcases? Some things may have to be shipped by UPS or by a moving company. However, having things moved by a moving company can take away a lot of extra money.

Travel nurses are some of the best shoppers at thrift stores! Take only the bare necessities and then go shopping when you get to your new assignment. If you are going to be living at an apartment complex and do not mind used stuff, watch for what is left beside the dumpsters.

Many treasures have been found there. Not that the items are "bad," but when others move from these complexes, you would be amazed at what they leave behind. Just like you, others do not want to drag around stuff, so they leave it behind.

On my first assignment, my husband and I found a vacuum cleaner and a futon bed. The lady who put them there came out of her apartment just about that time and asked us if we also wanted her television cabinet. Wow! The cabinet turned out to be a corner television cabinet made out of oak, with room for my son's video games below.

After making the thrift store rounds, then go to a discount store to purchase the rest of your necessities.

When you leave, you take the important and expensive stuff with you as much as possible, sell what you can, take it back to the thrift store for a tax credit, or set it back out at the dumpsters for the next traveler.

If you are moving to an extended stay or motel, things are much easier. They usually have pots, pans, and dishes. If not, go back to the thrift store and get a small and a large pot to cook with, and one or two dishes and cups. Do not forget to also get a microwave-safe cooking dish. Before you leave, make sure that your recruiter or housing supervisor tells you exactly what "furnished" will mean for that assignment.

If you are staying at a hotel or extended stay, necessity is a slow cooker. They will usually have a microwave already in place at the motel or extended stay. With a microwave and slow cooker, you can have hot meals ready when you come home from work.

If you're dragging or driving your home with you, you do not have as many things to "pack up," but you need to load the RV with the necessities before you add your other wants and needs of comfort. Included in your RV, you do not want to forget your coffee maker and slow cooker. It has also been my experience that we ladies cannot forget a bag—or two, or three—with our craft and sewing items. I have even been to a few travel trailers with sewing machines right next to their computer on the "dining" room table. Scrap-booking materials are also necessary for some travel nurses.

Be sure to pack your necessary nursing documents, such as your last tuberculosis test, your hepatitis C immunization records, and any other immunization records that your company required you to list on the forms that you sent in. Even though you probably sent them a copy, always have them available. Pack at least copies of your certificates, and carry your nursing license with you at all times. Be prepared to produce any other documents that human resources may ask for.

Be sure to call the place where you are supposed to stay and inquire as to whether all the necessary arrangements have been made. There is nothing worse than getting to a place and have them say, "We weren't expecting you." Make sure that the landlord of the apartment complex knows when you are expected to arrive, and arrange a tentative time to meet with him/her. I cannot stress enough the importance of getting all your housing arrangements guaranteed before you get to your assignment. This is where the great recruiter part comes in! Oh, and do not forget that wonderful recruiter's phone number.

The number one thing to do now enjoys a wonderful travel nursing assignment!

~*~

# Hungry For More Information?

## Check out our other travel nursing websites:

www.epsteinlarue.com

www.highwayhypodermics.com

# More Books by Epstein LaRue

*Highway Hypodermics: Travel Nursing 2017*

*Highway Hypodermics: Travel Nursing 2015*

*Highway Hypodermics: Travel Nursing 2012*

*Highway Hypodermics: On The Road Again*

*Highway Hypodermics: Travel Nursing 2007*

*Highway Hypodermics: Your Roadmap To Travel Nursing*

Made in the USA
Middletown, DE
15 October 2021

50382141R00040